AROMATHERAPY

An Informative Guide

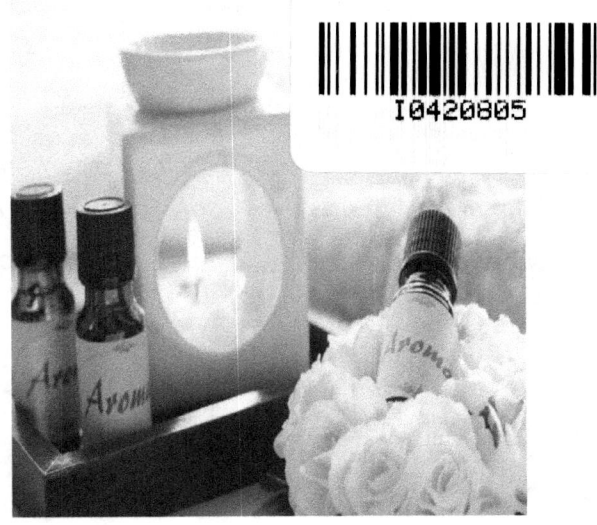

By

Meenakshi

Narang

Meenakshi Narang

Table of Contents

INTRODUCTION

Thanks for downloading this Book titled 'Aromatherapy: An Informative Guide'. This Book will guide you through the fundamentals of Aromatherapy - a holistic therapy that takes into account the physical and the mental well-being along with lifestyles and eating habits. This treatment involves addressing the imbalance in a patient especially with respect to cognitive function, mood or mental health. Aromatherapy massage is a branch of Aromatherapy that is known as *abhangaya* in Ayurveda which is a daily massage routine. Know in detail about origination and practicing of this alternate therapy and make most of its benefits!

Chapter 1: Beginning Of Aromatherapy

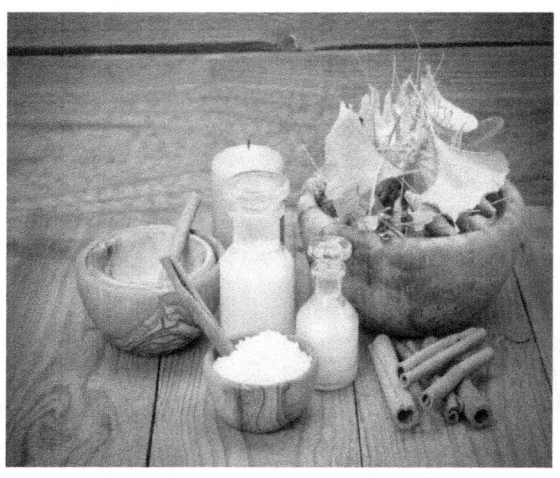

In India, the use of aromatic herbs can be traced through history, and was called *itr* meaning fragrance in Arabic. The history of itr is as old as the Indian civilization itself. The earliest instance of distillation of itr has been found in the Ayurvedic text called Charka Samhita. In 7th century AD, the Harshacharita mentions the use of fragrant agar wood oil.

In the modern era, the field of aromatherapy was established as a field of science in an accidental discovery by Rene Maurice Gatttefosse, a French chemist, who is responsible for coining the term 'Aromatherapy'. As reported, Gatttefosse suffered a burn injury while working in the lab. As a reflex, he dunked his hand in a tub of lavender oil, which was the nearest lying liquid. The burnt skin healed fast without any scarring.

This led him to research essential oils extensively. In 1937, Gatttefosse published the book titled Aromathérapie: Les Huiles Essentielles Hormones Vegetables. While this original work was in French, later an English translation titled as Aromatherapy was published; this is in print even today.

In ancient times essential oils were used for mystical experiences; however, now the effects of aromas have been scientifically studied. This has made possible a number of effective medications using aromatherapy.

For instance, Rosemary was used by Romans in religious or wedding ceremonies, in food and cosmetics, and the Egyptians used it as incense. Rosemary is known to be highly effective in stimulating hair growth, boosting mental activity, reducing pain and relieving respiratory problems. Thyme oil has also been found useful in the treatment of digestive and respiratory ailments.

Chapter 2: Medicinal Significance Of Ayurvedic Aromatherapy

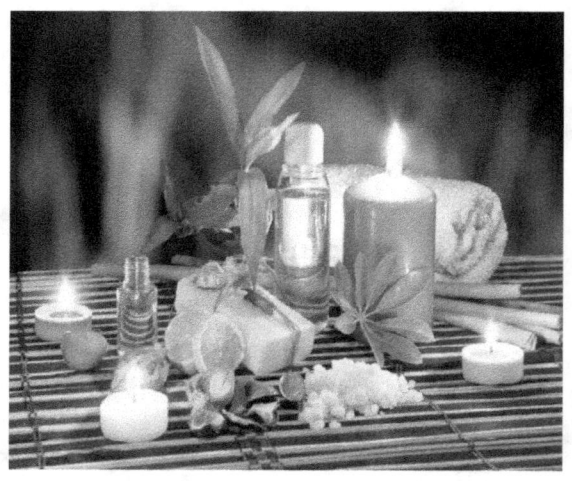

Aromatherapy believes that a healthy body is the result of a perfect unity between the physical and spiritual self. It takes into consideration lifestyle habits. The most extraordinarily striking part is that it gives the illness a chance to heal.

Ayurvedic Aromatherapy uses essential oils to set into motion it's larger objective of healing and recuperation and also ensures a healthy exchange between a proper diet, exercise, herbs, meditation, and yoga. All this in turn leads to the treatment of a number of diseases and prevention of yet more in number.

Aromatherapy is an example of a perfect coupling of medication and nature. It goes back to nature and uses natural ingredients for treatment of various problems and deformities. It indeed is a growing challenge to the monopoly of the conventional medicines used over time. This is the reason that an entire tourism industry is booming in countries like India, Egypt, and China, which specializes in Ayurvedic Aromatherapy.

The commonly used ingredients in Ayurvedic Aromatherapy include herbs and oils extracted from numerous plants, which have medicinal value. The oils extracted are supplied to the body in different ways that include adding them in bathing water, inhaling them or using them in diluted form.

Sharp scents are avoided, and warm scents are combined with calming oils. An amalgamation of oils extracted from camphor, cinnamon along with soothing ones like jasmine, rose, and sandalwood are considered apt.

It would not be wrong to categorize the technique as a holistic one that cares for everything. It renders great source of mental strength and goes a long way in providing a soothing effect on the mind. The ingredients and the techniques employed in Ayurvedic Aromatherapy are effective in reducing pain, fighting allergies, revitalizing the skin and providing a relaxed and calm mind.

There are a lot of stress-relieving oils that are used in Aromatherapy. These include lavender, bergamot and clary sage. Hand and foot massages with hazelnut or apricot oils are gaining popularity and are widely being employed just for shedding the tension and to gain peace and relieve. Aromatherapy goes a long way in detoxifying the body, which is extremely important. Using Aromatherapy oils for bathing, massaging and rubbing the neck and abdomen has the potential of relieving the body of unnecessary toxins.

Herbs like dandelion have a reputation of being excellent cleansers and detoxifiers.

Thyme thujanoll, eucalyptus radiata, ravintsara, tea tree oils are some of the oils that are effective in curing flu. These anti-viral oils can be used through massage or for intake and are extremely effective.

Not only this, a recent research has claimed that Aromatherapy could be effective in the treatment of serious diseases like dementia where patients sometimes lose their sense of memory and smell.

Chapter 3: Method Of Aromatherapy

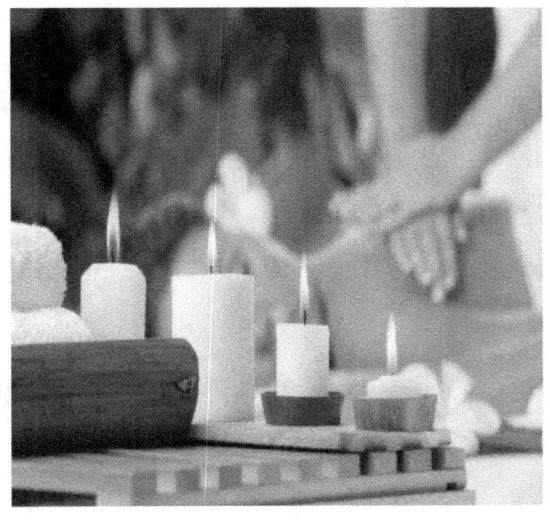

The process of smelling is a chemical one and is closely related to Aromatherapy, as a large part of Aromatherapy focuses on smell for its preventative measures. Vaporized odor molecules released by essential oils float in the air and then reach the nostrils and quickly dissolve in the mucus, which is the roof of each nostril.

The olfactory epithelium situated underneath the mucus paves a way for the molecules to reach the olfactory receptors that are special receptors and the neurons detect the odor. The odor formed there is transferred to the olfactory bulbs situated at the back of the nose.

The olfactory bulbs are of primary importance. This is so because they are home to the sensory receptors, which form a pivotal part in the brain. The message catalyzed by the essential oils aim to cure the patient of a particular disease. It then gets transmitted to the brain center and these in turn have a substantial impact on emotions, memories and other higher levels of the conscious.

In simple terms, the scent of certain oils and herbs has a soothing, calming effect and can cure certain illnesses. These herbs when used in the right manner, can help build immunity and also help fight against many illnesses.

The mechanism behind Aromatherapy is still not completely understood and requires a lot more work to uncover its full potential. However, the aromas induced by the essential oils have an influence on the brain and an impact on the limbic structure and it is assumed to have a desired effect.

Mode of Application

Ayurvedic Aromatherapy is quite diverse in its application and thereby can be made available through a number of means depending upon the individuals need and requirement. The three widely accepted modes of application are the topical application, direct inhalation, and aerial diffusion.

Aerial diffusion is similar to environmental fragrance. Its purpose is to fill a room with a natural fragrance. One could make use of certain simple methods and devices to carry out the diffusion effectively. Simple tissue diffusion is easy, convenient and easily transferable. It is very instrumental in a workplace or a public place as one could easily complete it by putting drops of aroma in a tissue and the aroma itself diffuses as one moves.

Steam diffusion, however, is a faster means of diffusing an aroma in a room. The steam helps to heat the oil and thereby bring about a faster diffusion of oils in the air. Candle diffusion also works for many. However, as the essential oils are flammable, so this method demands a lot of caution. The aroma is not long-lasting and sometimes, due to the heat, its effect might fade away faster.

Products for diffusion include lamp ring diffusers made of terracotta or brass. These are not expensive; rather they are efficient to carry out a desired purpose. Fan diffusers are available in the market, and they help to diffuse the aroma in the air. Electric heat diffusers are effective in spreading the fragrance in a larger area and are also more productive when it comes to thicker oils. Oil nebulizers can also be considered as one of the many options available in the market.

Direct inhalation is a means of disinfecting the respiratory system. It decreases congestion, increases and enables expectoration and also psychologically enhances one's moods and energies. Among the many advantages of direct inhalation are stimulation of the brain and immune system, mood enhancement, and relaxation.

In this method, the person in question is required to breathe the evaporating oil straight in. It could be done easily by placing a few drops of the essential oil on the palm and rubbing the hands. Place hands over the face are carefully protecting the eyes and after that the oil should be inhaled three to five times.

One could also inhale directly from the bottle by keeping it 6 to 8 inches away from the nose. It is soothing and imparts a calming effect. Inhalation is sometimes preferred over other methods especially in cases where the goal is weight loss, growth hormone secretion or even balancing emotions.

Topical application is manifested in baths, massages, compresses and the likes.

These, in fact, form the backbone of the popular perception of Ayurvedic Aromatherapy. Very commonly employed, these means are popularized a great deal by the spa centers and the emerging tourism and hospitality industry. The means employed in the topical application are said to ensure and facilitate a healthy blood circulation, pain relief and thereby restoring a stress-free life.

Hot compresses are no less than a blessing for people susceptible to migraine headaches, sore muscles, and sinus headaches. Peppermint oils, rosewood, and neroli, are recommended in this case. It follows a simple method that is to soak a piece of clothing in hot water, which has drops of the essential oil, and placing the cloth on the patient's head and repeating the process. Instant relief is guaranteed.

A hot bath not only provides relaxation but also relieves the mucus build-up in the lungs and at the same time replenishes the skin. Hot bath is used with the essential oils of sandalwood, rose, grapefruit and can be used solely for relaxing purposes or can even be used to heal skin allergies and disorders and relieve pain. It is said to improve lymph circulation and reduce the stress-levels.

Lemon, cedar wood, and rosemary are the perfect and most commonly used essential oils employed in massages. They are a great source of getting rid of tension and relieving pain and stress. Massages are the most commonly employed means of spreading the spark of Ayurvedic Aromatherapy. Carrier lotions assume importance in this case. The most commonly used lotions are almond, shea and cocoa butter blended with the essential oils to suit the purpose. These have physical and psychological benefits that can be experienced after a soothing bath.

The topical application would be more effective if the oils are used in a way to make them stay in longer contact with the skin. More effectively they are absorbed, more effective they would be in healing. The evaporation of the oils can be prevented by keeping it under a layer of synthetic-free lotion. This enhances penetration. Muscle injuries or injuries in bones and ligaments are more effectively dealt with the topical application. The topical method application also works quite well with acupressure.

These three are thereby only different methods to make full use of the bounties of Ayurvedic Aromatherapies. One could easily make a choice and pick the methodology of application best suited to the situation at hand.

Chapter 4: Materials Used For Aromatherapy

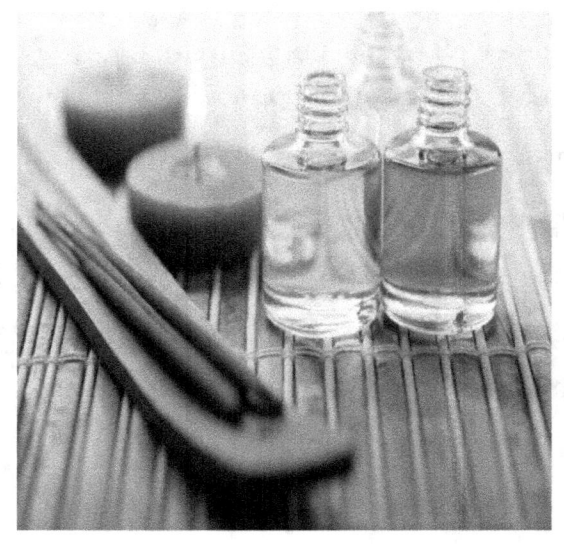

Like other medicinal divisions, Aromatherapy applies its ingredients and materials that help in the curing process. Materials employed for practicing and treating with Aromatherapy are as follows:

Essential oils

Essential oils first came into the commercial picture in 1920's, when Rene Maurice Gatttefosse, a French chemist had burned his hand in a laboratory explosion; he used lavender oil. Its antiseptic properties, which delineated from chemical ones, were quite helpful to heal his hand. This drew his attention towards the dermatological aspect of the lavender oil and consequently other oils too. While working in his family's perfume company, he got interested in the antiseptic value of these oils. Eventually, he coined the term Aromatherepie and published a book with the same name by 1937.

Later, other French doctors like Jean Valet would use these essential oils in the treatment of soldiers and sometimes to treat psychiatric patients despite much skepticism by other doctors. He continued the work of Gatttefosse in Aromatherapie. Essential oils, as against their chemical counterparts are seen to be more responsive and subtle, due to multiple properties that oil constitutes within itself. Chemical ones, on the contrary, carry within them usually a single property where their sole aim is to fix the problem since they are tailored to do so. Essential oils, on the contrary, have a balancing effect; their sole motive is more than treating a specific problem. It takes the idea of balancing from Ayurveda, which follow the principle of balance.

These same qualities are followed in case of Psychological imbalances such as depression, mood swings, hysteria. For long these have been considered as an excess of one of the humor. Considering this imbalanced state, these essential oils cater to the well being of the patient through their fragrance that gives a therapeutic effect to the mind. These are seen as better alternatives than conventional psychotropic drugs. Moreover, human contact while massaging, forms an important extension of Aromatherapy.

These oils have a property of readily being absorbed through the skin; they are used in cosmetics like lotions or used as compressors that are volatile essences that have a property of inhalation that soothes the mind, giving a sense of relaxation. By using them in lotions, these oils can be useful in the treatment of acne and eczema that promotes a healthy and beautiful complexion.

However, it is always advised to use prescribed essential oils and use them in right amounts by consulting an Aroma therapist since insufficient knowledge can lead to hazardous results.

Absolutes

As opposed to essential oils, which require steam distillation for preparation, absolutes on the contrary use the method of solvent extraction and enfleurage - a process that uses solid, odorless fats at room temperature in order to capture the fragrance of the plant. These processes are used especially in case of flower petals where there is a lesser risk of breaking, unlike distillation. The process of enfluerage yields a material known as 'pomade', which is a mixture of essential oils and fats. Solvent extraction produces a concrete of waxes, fats, essential oils and other plant materials. This pomade and concrete are treated with alcohol in order to extract the absolute.

This absolute that is produced is essential a highly concentrated, highly-aromatic, oily mixture. This process is usually run at low temperatures so as to avoid breakage of these petals. Since these have high aromatic and therapeutic effects, even a slight concentration of this absolute becomes sufficient. In case of rose absolutes, they solidify when kept at room temperatures, however, when they are held in the hand these liquefy.

Often, the usage of absolutes is avoided since it carries with itself a few traces of solvents, even after extraction from the concrete or pomade. These can be harmful; however sometimes these are used by Aroma therapists in low quantities.

Carrier oils

Commonly known as vegetable oils or base oils, carrier oils are used for diluting essential oils and absolute oils for topical application for massages and in

Aromatherapy. They absorb the essential oils into the skin. Unlike essential oils, they don't contain any concentrated aroma; however, some oils like olive oil have a mild smell.

These do not evaporate like essential oils, which are volatile. The carrier oils used should be as natural and unadulterated as possible. Maceration and Cold-pressing are the two main methods of producing carrier oils. These methods are as follows:

Cold pressed method: In this process one needs to make sure that the therapeutic acids and vitamins do not get destroyed. You need to avoid excessive heat for minimizing the changes in the innate properties of the oils.

Maceration: These carrier oils have added properties with respect to its production. In this method, parts of particular plants are cut and mixed with certain carrier oils like olive oil or sunflower oil. This mix is gently stirred for a certain span of time and then stored in a warm area. All the essential oils are then transferred into the carrier oil and then the macerated mix is carefully filtered, so that the excess plant material can be separated.

Considering the presence of a range of different carrier oils each with various therapeutic properties, the choice of appropriate oil will depend on the area that will be massaged, skin sensitivity, and the individual's requirements. Viscosity is a major consideration; for instance, grape seed oil is very thin while olive oil is much thicker. Sunflower and sweet almond have viscosities in between.

Herbal Distillates

These are hydrosols that are aqueous by-products of distillation, such as rosewater. These are suspensions of essential oils as well as water soluble components obtained by steam distillation of plants/herbs. These herbal distillates are used in flavoring, medicine, and skin care. These herbal distillates are also called floral water, hydrosol, and herbal water.

Although, the production of herbal distillates is similar to essential oils, however, the essential oil floats at the top of the distillate where it is removed, leaving the watery distillate as suspension. Initially known as the by-product of distillation, now these herbal distillates are considered an important by-product.

Most of the herbal waters contain diluted essential oils. These are very popular among cosmetics and toiletries makers. Ph value in the range of 5-6 is usually found to be suitable for skin facials. Other uses include room sprays and fresheners.
Production at high temperatures makes these hydrosols mildly acidic. This avoids bacterial growth. These should be kept refrigerated.

Infusions

The process of removing the flavors or chemical compounds from the plants into a solvent like water, alcohol or some oil is called infusion. In this method, it is required to allow the plant material to stay suspended inside the solvent for some time. The resultant liquid is called as the infusion.

For this process, plant materials used must be volatile and should dissolve the active ingredients in oil, water or alcohol. The plant materials are used as dry herbs, berries or flowers. The liquid (oil, water or alcohol) is boiled to the right temperature and then dispensed on the herb so that it seeps inside the solvent liquid. The liquid is either strained to remove the plants, or the herbs are separated from the liquid. The infusion is then refrigerated or bottled for further use.

The process is about 30 minutes long, as the mixture needs to cool down. The time required for preparation of this mixture also depends on its use. Various metal strainers or tea infusers maybe used in order to remove the left over material that was used in the infusion. These tea bags are used which have rich flavors and rich herbal content was providing the requisite need.

Phytoncides

Phytoncides are volatile antimicrobial chemical compounds that are derived from plants. Coined by Russian Biochemist, Dr. Boris P Tokin, Phytoncides mean, "something that is exterminated from the plant". As per Dr. Tokin, certain plants excrete active ingredients that prevent them from being eaten by insects and from rotting.

Some good examples of Phytoncides are spice, garlic, onion, oak tree, tea tree and pine tree. These volatile substances defend the plants from bacterial and fungal growth. For instance, each of these plants/herbs produces a unique phytoncide.

- Oak – greenery alcohol,
- Garlic-allicin and diallyl disulfide
- Sophora flavescent -sophoraflavanone G

- Pine - alpha-pinene, carene, myrcene

These are widely used in Russian, Chinese, and Ukrainian medicine. Other than Aroma therapy they are also used in veterinary medicines.

Chapter 5: Popular Oils

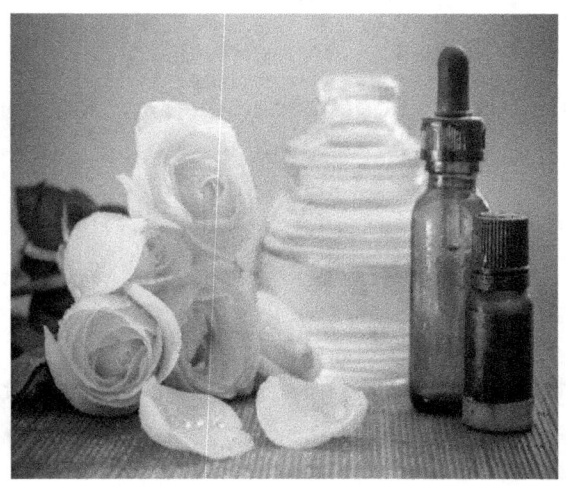

Aromatherapy employs a lot of different fragrant oils that have healing and soothing properties. Some of them are listed below.

Thyme Oil

Thyme oil has a sweet and strong herbal smell. It is extracted from steam or distillation of the fresh/partly dried flowering tops and leaves of the thyme plant. It was used in ancient times by the Greeks, the Romans, and the Egyptians for medicinal purposes.

The oil derives its name from the Greek word 'thymos' which means 'perfume' which is related to its use as incense in Greek temples. The Egyptians also used it in the embalming process.

Thyme oil is found to strengthen the nerves and enhance concentration and memory. It can help to overcome the feeling of exhaustion (in the Middle Ages it was given to knights for courage) and combats depression. It also fortifies the lungs and helps with a number of body ailments like colds, coughs, sore throats, laryngitis, catarrh, asthma, sinusitis, chills whooping cough and tonsillitis.

This oil has a warming effect on the area of application, and this can help with the problems of poor circulation, rheumatism, arthritis, gout, muscular aches, sprains and other sports injuries. It is also helpful for people suffering from anorexia, cellulite, obesity or edema and also in cases of scanty and irregular periods and leucorrhoea.

Thyme oil boosts the immune system and is very effective in fighting colds, flu, and other infectious diseases. It is very helpful for urethritis and cystitis as a urinary antiseptic.

Though essential oils have been observed to blend normally together quite well, Thyme oil blends particularly well with lemon, grapefruit, bergamot, rosemary, pine and lavender.

Peppermint Oil

A native to the Mediterranean, the pale yellow peppermint oil has a fresh and sharp, menthol-like smell. It is extracted from a perennial herb that has slight saw-like leaves and pink/mauve flowers. It is extracted from the plant's body (either fresh or partly dried) that is on the surface of the ground before flowering.

This herb has many species, and this might produce varieties of the oil with slight differences. Peppermint piperita is a hybrid of two such sub-species, spearmint (M. spicata) and watermint (M. aquatica). While it is cultivated in China and Japan since thousands of years, there is ample evidence of its use in a tomb in Egypt, dating back to almost 1000 BC.

Peppermint oil is excellent for several skin related problems like skin irritation, itchiness, skin redness due to inflammation (in which case the cooling effect of the oil on the skin helps).It is used for acne, dermatitis, scabies, ringworm and pruritus and also for relieving itching or sunburn.

Peppermint oil provides the cure for a range of problems related to the digestive system. This is because it fuels the gall bladder and enhances the discharge of bile, thereby healing several digestive problems.

Benzoin, lemon, rosemary, lavender, marjoram, and eucalyptus are some of the oils that blend well with peppermint oil.

Lavandula Oil

An extract of LavandulaAugustifolia, Lavandula oil, is more popularly known as lavender oil. This oil has a clear color along with watery viscosity. It has a fresh aroma and has been used in bath routines since the ancient times among the Romans.

Lavandula oil has a very soothing effect on the skin, and it is effective enough to heal minor wounds. It revitalizes and even tones the skin and is used for almost different types of skin issues like oily skin, acne, burns, boils, insect bites, lice, and stings.

It also works as an insect repellant when applied and can relax the nerves, to relieve tension, panic, depression, hysteria and is also used to cure migraines, headaches, and insomnia.

It helps with several ailments related to the digestive system (vomiting, nausea, colic and flatulence); and the respiratory system (asthma, colds, throat infections, halitosis, whooping coughs, laryngitis and bronchitis).

Lavandula oil is also beneficial in relieving pain in cases of arthritis, rheumatism, lumbago and muscular pains, especially those related to sporting activities.

Lavender oil particularly blends well with other oils like pine, geranium, all kinds of citrus oils, clary sage and cedar wood.

Jasmine Oil

Jasmine essential oil is extracted from the white-star shaped flowers of the jasmine shrubs that are evergreen, fragile creepers that can grow up to 10 meters. It is picked at night when its aroma is at its peak. Jasmine oil has been used for medicinal purposes since the ancient times by the Chinese, Indians, and the Arabians.

Because of its soothing floral smell, it produces a feeling of euphoria, confidence, and optimism. It soothes the nerves, overcomes the feelings of depression and revitalizes and restores energy. Again because of its deeply calming nature, jasmine oil helps with a number of sexual problems such as premature ejaculation, impotency, and frigidity (hence, its ancient use is as of aphrodisiac).

This oil is non-toxic, non-irritant and also non-sensitizing. Thus, it does not show any side-effects. The therapeutic properties of jasmine oil which determines its various applications are an aphrodisiac, antiseptic, anti-depressant, anti-spasmodic, expectorant, cicatrisant, parturient, galactagogue, uterine and sedative.

Jasmine oil is also beneficial in facilitating delivery during childbirth. It strengthens the contractions thereby hastening the birth and also relieves the labor pain. It is also effective in curing post-natal depression. It benefits the new mother during the lactation period by promoting the flow of breast milk.

Jasmine oil tones skin increases elasticity and is often used to assist with stretch marks and to reduce scarring.

Jasmine Oil has a very beneficial effect on ailments related to the respiratory system. It soothes irritating coughs and helps with laryngitis and hoarseness.

The essential oils that Jasmine oil blends particularly well with are the rose, bergamot, sandalwood and all citrus oils.

Chapter 6: Using Ayurvedic Aromatherapy For Common Ailments

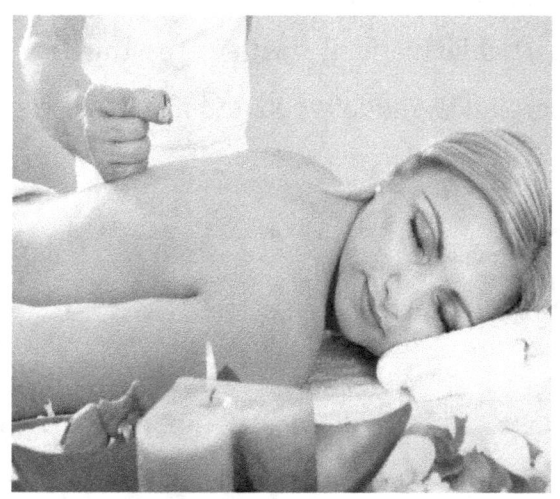

Acupuncture

Patients were suffering from chronic pain (for example, after surgery) usually look for alternative or complementary treatments. Therapies, such as Acupuncture, Aromatherapy and

Acupressure have been seen as efficient in controlling chronic pain.

Acupuncture involves the stimulation of specific acu points in the body by the application of pressure, heat, laser or penetration of thin needles. Treating directly the reflex points in the pain areas simultaneously promotes the well-being of the nervous system by increasing its variability, thereby indicating the ability to adapt to variable external conditions.

Combining the knowledge of Acupuncture and Aromatherapy, there is a separate form of therapy often regarded as 'Acu-Aromatherapy'. Acu-Aromatherapy is the use of particular blends of therapeutic grade essential oils to stimulate acupuncture points. It may / may not involve the use of needles.

Oils used in Aromatherapy can be absorbed through the pores in the skin or the nose. Oils are easily sensed by the receptors in the nose, which carry it to the brain with the help of neurons. Often the oils are applied to the palms of the hand or the bottom of the feet from where they are absorbed into the blood stream in less than five minutes.

Acu-Aromatherapy brings the best of both healing practices. Acupuncture with Aromatherapy enhances the stimulation of the acu-points, speeding up the process of healing.

Acne

Acne is one of the worst skin condition faced by a majority of the population across the world. The problem of acne is typically associated with clogged skin pores. When the skin pores and follicles are blocked due to dirt, proper secretion of natural skin oils is blocked, and it builds up under the skin. This provides a fertile ground for bacteria to multiply.

It causes acne that is also linked to hormonal fluctuations and, therefore, is more common among teenagers.

Aromatherapy not just clears the skin but does it by helping the management of the very underlying problems that cause acne. They regulate the oil production by the oil glands under the skin, balance hormones and regulate fluctuations, reduce stress, and improve the complexion.

This is why Aromatherapy is the ideal treatment for acne problems like pimples, blemishes, and other types of skin eruptions. This is the reason even chemical products in the market claim to have been inspired by an Ayurvedic formula containing essential oils such as eucalyptus oil, lemon or lavender.

Essential oils are also effective in fighting off bacteria from the acne affected region. Salt along with essential oil compress is a good remedy for acne. Essential oils have a skin-drying and antiseptic quality. Eucalyptus, geranium, cedar wood, sandalwood, lemongrass, frankincense, lavender, tea tree, clary sage, juniper berry and lemon are he best essential oils. These oils can be diluted in an aloe vera or witch hazel base gel. Witch hazel is especially good in balancing oily skin because of the presence of alcohol in its composition.

Addiction

Lately, Aromatherapy has become a popular therapeutic practice in treating the withdrawal symptoms during a drug addiction treatment. Though varying according to the addiction of drug, withdrawal symptoms include sleep disturbances, restlessness, irritability, and anxiety. Essential oils used in

Aromatherapy help to create an emotional balance, promoting a sense of calm by reducing the feelings of stress. The result of this is a considerable reduction in several withdrawal symptoms.

Aromatherapy is mostly used as an adjunct to support the traditional addiction treatment methods. Aromatherapy, when combined with massage therapy, considerably improves the therapeutic value of the latter. It produces a greater sense of holistic well-being because of an increased sense of relaxation and healing of pain.

Below listed are some of the Aromatherapy essential oils that are especially beneficial in treatment of withdrawal symptoms:

Anise Aromatherapy: Anise curbs cravings for chocolate or sugary items that are often experienced by those fighting alcohol addictions. It also relieves stress and induces better sleep and provides relaxation.

Chamomile Aromatherapy: Chamomile has been traditionally regarded as an antidepressant. It helps to relieve suppressed anger and thus provides relaxation and aids sleep. It is also helpful in decreasing addictive cravings.

Frankincense Aromatherapy: Frankincense induces spirituality, clears perception, and leads to higher states of consciousness. It encourages a kind of optimism and also helps in a release from the past. It is also effective in combating cravings for sugar or sedatives.

Lavender Aromatherapy: Lavender provides relief from lethargy and exhaustion due to work, calms the nerves, thus helping during the withdrawal phase. It also reduces cravings for alcohol.

Fennel Aromatherapy: Fennel also helps in dispelling cravings for chocolate, alcohol and sugar, common during the withdrawal phase.

Alzheimer's disease and other forms of dementia

Yes, it may sound quite surprising but it is true, Aromatherapy plays an important role in treating dementia and Alzheimer's disease to a great extent. People were suffering from Alzheimer's disease or other forms of dementia frequently experience states of agitation that makes them a challenge to their family or caregivers.

Traditional medication involves the use of strong tranquilizers that suppress such feelings of agitation, but it is accompanied by partial or full unconsciousness of the patient. Thus, Ayurvedic Aromatherapy becomes an important form of alternative medication in which essential oils are applied to the patients through methods like massage, direct inhalation, bath, ambient diffusion, etc.

Different essential oils show varying properties. Some popular and easily available essential oils used in the medication of dementia include:

Lavender: It is an antidepressant that calms the nerves and balances strong emotions. It is also good for insomnia, thus, promoting better sleep and a better overall mood.

Rosemary: Rosemary essential oil stimulates body and mind, creating a feeling of emotional well-being. It also improves the cognitive performance of the mind in its accuracy and also in terms of speed.

Peppermint: When used in the morning, it boosts appetite. It stimulates the mind and calms the nerves. It is also helpful in keeping a check on absent-mindedness caused by dementia.

Lemon Balm: It induces a feeling of calmness and relaxation and is very effective in cases of anxiety and insomnia.

Chapter 7 - Preparation Of Essential Oil: Solvent Extraction Method

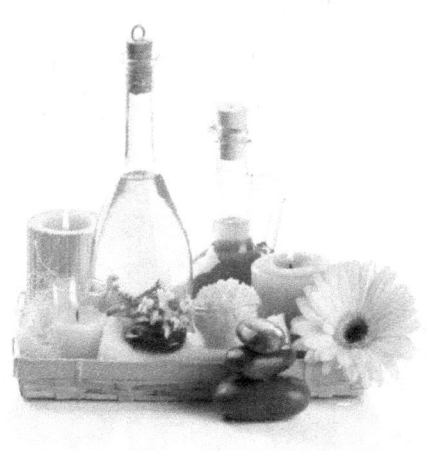

Different categories of essential oils are -

• Flowers – Possible sources are lavender, rose, jasmine, marigold, and frangipani etc.

- Herbs – Possible sources are basil, peppermint, thyme, marjoram, lemon balm, etc.

- Spices – Possible sources are coriander, nutmeg, cumin, cloves, cinnamon, etc.

After collecting the sources, the following materials will be required:

- The flower or herb that is used

- High proof alcohol like 120 proof Vodka or Neutral grain spirit

- Canning jars made from clear glass

- Freezer

- Amber glass bottles. A dropper shall be required for getting essential oils in the bottle.

- Strainer, especially one coated with porcelain

- Cheese cloth

- Glass bowl

- Kitchen items like spoons and bowls

Procedure

➢ After deciding on an herb or flower, you need to understand its highest fragrance level. Flowers picked in the morning are the most appropriate, because as the day descends the scent of the flowers gets dissipated by the sun. Flowers like moonflower or evening primrose, which bloom at night, should be ideally picked after sunset. The part with the highest scent is required, which can either be petals or the center. The intensity of the smell denotes the oil content in the plant. When using some scented plants like peppermint, it is advisable to test both the mature leaves and the newly bloomed leaves and avoid the stem as it may turn the batch sour and change the scent. For specific plants like chamomile you can gather different scents from the leaves and the flowers.

➢ When using plants, you need to remember that only small quantities of scent can be gathered. For home made essential oils, this plant essence could be in drops, in contrast to commercial producers.

➢ Dry the chosen plant material. However, the idea is that you dry the water content in the plant and not the plant in itself. You can use a dehydrator till the plant begins to fade; you can also place the plant between absorbent papers for a few hours and let it soak the water. The time shall vary since every plant is different, and the climatic condition plays an important part in drying.

➤ Place the plant in a canning jar and pour the spirit, so that the plant material is just about covered. Seal it and shake it for around 3 minutes. Leave the mixture in room temperature and away from sunlight in a cool dark place.

➤ Shake the mixture well about 2 to 3 times a day. The mixture should rest till the time the color starts to fade from the plant that usually takes 3-4 days.

➤ Strain the mixture out of the alcohol carefully and then wrap the plant material in a linen or cheese cloth and squeeze it tight so that every drop of liquid gets utilized. In order to repeat this process, the same alcohol may be used

➤ In the end, pour the alcohol into the canning jar, seal the jar and keep aside. Carefully observe a separation happening, a scummy part will float at the top or may go right at the bottom, whereas the Neutral Grain Spirits rest at the bottom of the jar. Place the jar in the freezer finally.

➢ Alcohol placed in the freezer does not freeze, on the contrary, essential oils and the scummy part will.

➢ Before the concoction thaws, take a linen or cheese cloth in a jar. Then take another clean jar secure it with a linen or cheese cloth at the opening so that a large dip forms at the mouth of the jar. Take another glass bowl and a typical amber oil bottle. Use a spoon and a dropper too.

➢ Since the scummy layer is either on the bottom or the top, follow either of the steps:

➢ If the layer is at the top, scoop the scrummy mass using a spoon and keep it inside a glass bowl (use a cheese cloth).

Do not scoop the other clear but colored essential oil. Pour the alcohol from the freezer in the jar with the cheese cloth. In case small frozen particles are caught in the linen or cheese cloth, remove them. If there are any particles of essential oils in the jar, scoop them out as well.

➢ If the scrummy mass is at the base of the jar, use a cheese cloth to pour the unfrozen alcohol in to the canning jar. Scoop away the frozen bits from the cheese cloth. Scoop out any frozen essential oils from the scrummy mass or from inside the jar.

➢ After collecting the scrummy mass, drain the thawed oil through the cheese cloth; however do not squeeze it. The drained part is the plant material

➢ The essential oils that are gathered in the white bowl can be transferred into the amber bottle with the dropper.

➢ In the similar fashion, you can store the alcohol into another jar. Place it in the freezer and let it freeze once again. When you take it out, only the essential oils will be frozen so that the collection will be much easier.

➢ This alcohol holds medicinal properties, which is also tincture. In tincture oil, the oil is not removed.